ACTIVE RELEASE

TECHNIQUES

A Complete Guide For Unlocking The
Body's Potential From Tension To
Liberation

WALTER ZYAIRE

DISCLAIMER

The information in this book is intended only for general informational purposes; it should not be used in lieu of professional advice or medical care. Since the author is not licensed to practice therapy, the information offered should not be used in place of the expertise, judgment, or guidance of qualified mental health or medical professionals. Readers are encouraged to consult therapists, medical specialists, or other qualified authorities regarding their particular situation and needs. The publisher and author disclaim all liability for any actions or decisions taken by readers based on the information in this book. Results may vary from person to person and this book's approaches, procedures, and strategies may not be suitable in all circumstances. Considering unique situations and consulting a qualified expert are essential when choosing the right course of action. Neither the publisher nor the author recommend or guarantee the efficacy of any therapy or treatment that is indicated in this book. Because the information is based on the author's research and understanding at the time of publishing, it could not reflect the most recent developments or practices in the treatment area. The publisher and the author both disclaim all liability for the accuracy, completeness, or use of the material in this book. Readers bear full responsibility for the decisions and actions they choose in light of the information presented in this book.

TABLE OF CONTENTS

ABOUT THE BOOK

Active Release Techniques (ART) is an extensive manual that explores the complexities of soft tissue therapy. It provides a deep comprehension of the mechanics of the human body and the utilization of specific procedures to improve function. This book is a useful resource for athletes, healthcare professionals, and anybody looking to maximize physical well-being since it can effectively bridge the gap between academic understanding and actual application.

The book's goal is made evident in the introduction, which also highlights the importance of ARTs in treating a range of ailments. It provides a thoughtful synopsis of ART and emphasizes the many advantages that result from implementing it in medical procedures. Through this method of laying the foundation, readers can see why ART is essential to the field of soft tissue therapy.

The book's later sections are organized methodically, starting with a thorough examination of the anatomy, physiology, and significance of soft tissues in the body's mechanics. The basic knowledge explains the concept, principles, and crucial role that tension and compression play in treatments, setting the basis for an understanding of the fundamentals of Active Release Techniques.

This book's overview of common illnesses handled by ART is one of its standout features. Looking at soft tissue injuries, repetitive strain injuries, sports-related injuries, and postural dysfunctions, goes beyond a general approach. By focusing on particular cases, the book turns into a valuable resource for medical professionals looking for tailored answers for a range of clinical circumstances.

A practical turn is taken in the hands-on procedures portion when particular ART protocols for the upper, lower, and spine are presented. This section improves the reader's capacity to use ART in practical situations with the help of case studies. In addition, the book promotes a holistic approach to healthcare by highlighting patient education, cooperation with other medical experts, and the incorporation of ART into rehabilitation programs.

The book's depth and breadth come from advanced ART applications, research and evidence supporting ART, training and certification procedures, and upcoming trends and developments. As such, it's a comprehensive resource for practitioners at all levels. The book presents itself as a cutting-edge resource in the field of soft tissue therapy by compiling the most recent research findings, cutting-edge technologies, and changing practices.

Essentially, the book on Active Release Techniques is a thorough guide that improves the comprehension and utilization of soft tissue therapy, rather than just a handbook. The methodical approach, practical methods, and integration of contemporary advancements and trends render it an invaluable tool for healthcare practitioners seeking to provide efficient, evidence-based treatment.

CHAPTER ONE

OVERVIEW OF ACTIVE RELEASE TECHNIQUES

THE ACTIVE RELEASE TECHNIQUES (ART)

An advanced and successful manual therapy method called Active Release Techniques (ART) is used to treat a range of musculoskeletal disorders. ART was created by chiropractor Dr. P. Michael Leahy and has become well-known for its distinct approach to treating soft tissue disorders and injuries.

The basic tenet of ART is that soft tissues such as tendons, ligaments, and overworked muscles can form adhesions that impair their range of motion and cause pain. As a result, ART uses a combination of carefully administered tension, movement, and patient-specific procedures to dissolve these adhesions and give the afflicted tissues their normal function again.

The interactive, hands-on aspect of art is one of its defining characteristics. Practitioners assess the texture, tightness, and mobility of muscles with their hands to spot any aberrant adhesions or tension in certain locations. They then apply carefully directed tension using a methodical technique as the patient actively moves the injured body part through a predetermined range of motion. A customized and focused treatment that meets each patient's specific needs is made possible by the practitioner-patient dynamic interaction that sets ART apart from passive therapies.

THE ADVANTAGES OF INCLUDING ART IN MEDICAL PROCEDURES

Active Release Techniques have many advantages for both healthcare providers and patients when used in their professions. Its capacity to successfully cure a variety of ailments, such as but not limited to muscular strains, tendinitis, ligament injuries, and nerve entrapments, is one of its main benefits.

Because of its adaptability, ART is a useful tool for medical professionals like physical therapists, chiropractors, and sports medicine specialists.

Moreover, ART treats the underlying cause of musculoskeletal problems in addition to its symptoms. ART delivers long-term relief and improves general biomechanics by breaking down adhesions and enhancing the flexibility and function of soft tissues. This proactive approach promotes a holistic awareness of the interdependence of the body's numerous systems and is in line with the increasing emphasis on preventative healthcare.

One further important advantage of ART is that it helps quicken the healing process. Patients frequently report less discomfort and quicker healing times as a result of enhanced range of motion and the restoration of appropriate tissue function. This enables a quicker return to training and competition, which can be very helpful for sportsmen and people leading active lifestyles.

ART is also well-known for being non-invasive, making it a good substitute for or in addition to more intrusive therapies. Patients value that ART is a low-risk treatment with few adverse effects because it doesn't require surgery or medication. This is consistent with the larger trend in healthcare toward patient-centered, conservative methods that give priority to the body's healing mechanisms.

A dynamic and successful strategy for treating musculoskeletal problems is the integration of Active Release Techniques into healthcare procedures. With its capacity to treat a wide range of problems and its hands-on, patient-specific approach, ART provides a proactive and comprehensive option for both patients and practitioners. With its focus on regaining normal tissue function, speeding up recovery, and offering a non-invasive substitute, ART is positioned to be a useful instrument in the changing field of manual therapy and rehabilitation.

CHAPTER TWO

COMPREHENDING THE MECHANICS OF THE BODY

PHYSIOLOGY AND ANATOMY

The smooth operation of the human body's many systems is essential to its intricate functioning, and anatomy and physiology provide the foundation for comprehending this intricate machinery. Anatomy is the study of the organs, tissues, and systems that make up the body. It offers a guide to the complex web of interconnected parts. Physiology, on the other hand, reveals the mechanisms that support life by concentrating on the dynamic activities and functions that take place within these systems.

AN OVERVIEW OF THE MUSCULAR SYSTEM

The muscular system is essential to the body's mechanics because it produces heat, maintains posture, and allows for movement. There are three different kinds of muscles in this system: cardiac, smooth, and skeletal. Voluntary actions, including walking and lifting objects, are made possible by skeletal muscles, which are affixed to bones through tendons. Internal organ walls contain smooth muscles, which regulate involuntary processes like digestion.

The heart's unique cardiac muscles guarantee that blood flows continuously. The overall mechanical efficiency of the body is attributed to the synchronization and synergy between different muscle types.

Muscles are essential for performing both fine and gross motor abilities because they work on the concept of contraction and relaxation. The nervous system is involved in this dynamic interplay because coordinated motions are produced when inputs from the brain cause muscular contractions. The delicate balance between the agonist and antagonist muscles is what makes this technique so effective; it guarantees a smooth and regulated range of motion.

THE VALUE OF CONNECTIVE TISSUES

The body's soft tissues, which include muscles, ligaments, tendons, and fascia, play a major role in its mechanical integrity. Muscles, consisting of contractile fibers, produce the force required for motion. Tendons provide force and promote joint movement by joining muscles to bones. In turn, ligaments give support by joining one bone to another. Connective tissue called fascia surrounds and divides muscles and organs to create a supporting framework.

The significance of soft tissues is not limited to biomechanics. Strains, sprains, and tears are among the ailments that can occur to soft tissues and impair the body's mechanical functions. To keep these tissues healthy and resilient, proper maintenance is essential. This includes stretching, strengthening activities, and getting enough sleep. Furthermore, soft tissue health influences posture, flexibility, and the avoidance of musculoskeletal problems, all of which are linked to overall well-being.

Ultimately, exploring the complexities of anatomy and physiology reveals the wonders of the human body's workings. The intricate relationship between muscles and soft tissues is crucial because the muscular system, with its many parts, coordinates movement and function. Understanding the importance of these components enhances our knowledge of the mechanics of the body and highlights the necessity of holistic care to preserve optimum health and functionality.

CHAPTER THREE

PRINCIPLES OF ACTIVE RELEASE METHODS

ART'S GUIDING PRINCIPLES AND PHILOSOPHY

Targeting soft tissue dysfunction, Active Release Techniques (ART) is a manual therapy strategy intended to treat a variety of musculoskeletal problems. Fundamentally, the application of ART is shaped by a set of values and a unique philosophy. The underlying idea is that muscles, ligaments, fascia, and nerves are all interconnected parts and issues with one might arise from issues with others. The holistic approach of ART is based on this interconnectivity.

The foundation of alternative medicine (ART) is the idea that, given the correct circumstances, the body may naturally heal itself. ART practitioners diagnose and treat specific soft tissue dysfunctions to promote this healing process that occurs naturally. In addition to manual treatment, they stress the value of patient participation in the healing process and promote active engagement through exercises and lifestyle changes.

TENSION AND COMPRESSION'S ROLE

In the context of ART, tension and compression are crucial. The therapy acknowledges that a variety of reasons, including overuse, trauma, or poor posture, can cause soft tissues to form adhesions, scar tissue, and tightness. Tension is the state of stress and strain that occurs in muscles and connective tissues, whereas compression is the process of applying pressure to particular regions. To remove adhesions and restore normal movement patterns, ART practitioners precisely compress and tense the targeted tissues with their hands.

Another important idea in ART is trigger points, which you must recognize and handle by having a thorough understanding of their role in tension and compression. Localized locations of tension and soreness in the muscles that can radiate pain to other parts of the body are known as trigger points. ART professionals are taught to palpate and use manual examination to locate these trigger points. By using particular compression and tension methods on these trigger points, practitioners aim to enhance blood flow, relieve stress, and return the damaged muscles and surrounding tissues to normal function.

LOCATING THE POINTS OF TRIGGERING

A mix of expert palpation and patient discussion is required to identify trigger sites. To identify regions of dysfunction, practitioners evaluate the tension, mobility, and texture of tissues. They also depend on the patient's feedback, wherein the patient may report trigger point-related pain patterns or sensations. Because the therapy may be customized to the patient's specific condition, this participatory procedure enables a more effective and individualized application of ART.

The ART concept and guiding principles emphasize how interrelated the body's soft tissues are and how crucial it is to promote the body's natural healing process. In the hands of ART practitioners, tension and compression are essential tools that allow them to locate trigger points and apply precise manual procedures to address them. In the field of musculoskeletal therapy, this all-encompassing strategy combined with patient involvement characterizes the essence of Active Release Techniques.

CHAPTER FOUR

COMMON ISSUES THAT ART ADDRESSES

SOFT TISSUE INJURIES

These injuries cover a wide spectrum of ailments affecting the body's connective tissues, including muscles, tendons, ligaments, and other tissues. These injuries can arise from several different things, such as strain, trauma, or overuse.

Targeted manual manipulation is the method used to treat soft tissue injuries in the context of Active Release Techniques (ART). ART practitioners assess soft tissue movement, tightness, and texture with their hands to spot adhesions or other limitations.

Releasing tension and enhancing the functioning of impacted tissues is the aim, leading to an increased range of motion, increased flexibility, and less pain.

REPETITIVE STRAIN INJURIES (RSIS)

RTIs are frequently brought on by overusing or repeatedly using a certain body part, which can cause pain, discomfort, and malfunction. People who participate in occupations that require repetitive motions or extended periods in the same posture are frequently affected by these injuries. By focusing on the particular muscles and soft tissues implicated, ART aims to treat RSIs. To release tension and dissolve adhesions, practitioners use precise movements that promote better blood flow and faster healing. ART seeks to relieve pain and stop more damage by targeting the underlying causes of RSIs, allowing patients to resume their activities with a lower chance of recurrence.

SPORTS-RELATED AILMENTS

From muscle strains to ligament sprains and joint ailments, athletes commonly sustain a variety of injuries connected to their particular sports.

Sports-related injury prevention and rehabilitation are greatly aided by the use of active release techniques. Adhesions or scar tissue that may form as a result of trauma or repetitive strain from sports activities are identified and treated by ART practitioners. Through addressing these problems, ART seeks to help the athlete heal by restoring optimal strength, flexibility, and function. Adding ART to pre- and post-event routines can also help athletes in a variety of sports prevent injuries and improve their overall performance.

POSTURAL DYSFUNCTIONS

Defining imbalances or anomalies in the body's alignment, postural dysfunctions frequently result in pain, discomfort, and diminished functionality. Several things, such as extended periods of sitting, muscular imbalances, or prior injuries, can cause poor posture. By concentrating on the impacted soft tissues, Active Release Techniques provide a tailored approach to alleviate postural dysfunctions.

To promote improved alignment and muscular balance, practitioners relieve adhesions and stiffness using targeted motions and pressure. ART seeks to decrease related discomfort, improve posture, and improve total musculoskeletal function by combining manual treatment with remedial exercises. With this method, people can prevent the recurrence of dysfunction in their regular activities and preserve improved posture.

CHAPTER FIVE

PRACTICAL METHODS

PARTICULAR ART PROTOCOLS

A manual treatment method called Active Release Technique (ART) is used to treat soft tissue injuries and enhance musculoskeletal function. Particular ART methods are designed to precisely target different body parts. To break up scar tissue, remove adhesions, and regain optimal range of motion, these procedures combine pressure and movement. Professionals go through specific training to become proficient in these procedures and use them wisely.

TECHNIQUES FOR THE UPPER BODY

A variety of upper body treatments known as ART are used to treat ailments like carpal tunnel syndrome, tennis elbow, and shoulder impingement. The medical professional locates particular tendons, ligaments, or muscles that can be injured or restricted.

They try to relieve stress and encourage tissue repair by moving the patient and applying pressure with their hands. To assess and treat the complex network of muscles and connective tissues in the neck, shoulders, arms, and hands, upper body methods frequently use a methodical approach.

TECHNIQUES FOR THE LOWER BODY

In ART, lower body treatments are mostly used to treat problems with the hips, knees, ankles, and feet. These methods are intended to alleviate pain and dysfunction resulting from plantar fasciitis, patellar tendinitis, and iliotibial band syndrome.

The practitioner applies tension and directs the patient via precise motions using their hands to find and manipulate particular soft tissue structures. This method aids in the breakdown of scar tissue, enhances blood flow, and helps the lower extremities return to normal function.

TECHNIQUES FOR THE SPINE

Target issues affecting the neck, mid-back, and lower back using ART treatments for the spine. A thorough examination of the soft tissues around the vertebrae is a necessary part of spinal procedures, whether one is treating facet joint dysfunction, herniated discs, or sciatica. Using patient motions to increase therapy effectiveness, practitioners apply tension and compression to the afflicted areas with their hands. The goals of spinal procedures in ART are to reduce pain, increase range of motion, and reestablish the musculoskeletal system's equilibrium.

CASE STUDIES AND THEIR USE

Case studies are essential for illustrating the usefulness and effectiveness of ART treatments. These real-world examples demonstrate the use of particular approaches to various musculoskeletal problems. Practitioners frequently exchange knowledge about how assessments are made, how treatment plans are created, and what results each patient has received. These case studies offer a deeper knowledge of the technique's adaptability and effectiveness in a range of clinical circumstances, making them an invaluable resource for both seasoned ART practitioners and those just starting.

Active Release Technique protocols provide focused methods to target particular body parts, such as the spine, upper and lower extremities, and other areas. The manual methods used in ART are designed to break up scar tissue, loosen adhesions, and get the musculoskeletal system back to working optimally. Case examples from real-world situations highlight how these procedures can be used in practice and how they can aid in patients' overall rehabilitation and well-being.

CHAPTER SIX

INCLUDING ART IN PRACTICE

INCLUDING ART IN PROGRAMS FOR REHABILITATION

A comprehensive strategy that goes beyond conventional therapy techniques is provided by including art in rehabilitation programs since it acknowledges the inextricable link between creative expression and general well-being. Using art in rehabilitation settings enables people to participate in a creative process that can improve their recovery's cognitive, emotional, and physical components.

When used effectively, art therapy promotes communication and self-expression, which is especially beneficial for patients who have trouble verbalizing their experiences. This integration is a therapeutic approach that encourages healing by artistic discovery rather than just an aesthetic addition.

WORKING TOGETHER WITH OTHER MEDICAL EXPERTS

Working together with other medical professionals is crucial to providing patients with a thorough and multidisciplinary approach. Physiotherapists, psychiatrists, art therapists, and rehabilitation professionals collaborate through art to bridge disparate therapeutic vantage points. The combination of several areas of knowledge enables customized interventions to meet the needs of each patient, resulting in a comprehensive and unique rehabilitation strategy.

By merging the skills of several healthcare disciplines, this partnership improves the efficacy of interventions, improving patient outcomes and promoting a more holistic healing environment.

PATIENT EMPOWERMENT AND EDUCATION

Empowerment and education of patients are essential elements of effective rehabilitation programs.

By offering a real and visual medium for the explanation of difficult medical concepts, treatment methods, and recovery expectations, art is a potent educational tool. Visual aids, including artistic depictions or anatomical drawings, help patients grasp concepts more clearly and encourage health literacy and well-informed decision-making.

Moreover, including patients in artistic endeavors gives them a sense of empowerment as it increases their self-efficacy and sense of control over their healing process. People can regain control over their bodies and emotions through artistic expression, which has a favorable effect on their general well-being.

Realizing the therapeutic potential of art extends beyond its aesthetic value is essential to incorporating it into rehabilitation programs.

When healthcare professionals work together, the multifaceted aspects of patient care are improved, leading to a more customized and holistic approach.

Educating patients through the arts not only improves comprehension but also gives them the confidence to take an active role in their healing. Thus, the addition of art changes rehabilitation into an expressive and active path toward overall well-being.

CHAPTER SEVEN

ADVANCED APPLICATIONS FOR ART

USING ART TO IMPROVE PERFORMANCE

Applications of Advanced Adaptive Resonance Theory (ART) go beyond typical realms of problem-solving to include a variety of fields like performance enhancement.

By adjusting neural networks' stability and plasticity, artificial reinforcement learning (ART) is being used more and more in the fields of sports and athletics to maximize human performance. Because ART is adaptable, it can dynamically adapt to an athlete's changing skill set, allowing for customized training plans that focus on particular areas for growth. Superior athletic accomplishments are facilitated by ART, which continuously adjusts to each person's performance indicators. This makes the enhancement process more effective and efficient.

STRATEGIES FOR PREHABILITATION

Prehabilitation programs emphasize preventative efforts to lower the chance of injury or degeneration, and they offer a proactive approach to treatment. Prehabilitation in the context of ART refers to using adaptive learning algorithms to identify and correct possible physiological system imbalances or deficits in a patient. Through the examination of biomechanical data and individual features, ART can create prehabilitation plans that emphasize strengthening weak areas, increasing joint stability, and boosting resilience overall. This proactive strategy not only reduces the chance of injury but also promotes maximum physical health and functionality, which enhances long-term well-being.

PROLONGED UPKEEP AND INJURY AVOIDANCE

An essential component of ART applications is long-term maintenance and injury prevention, particularly in domains where continuous performance is crucial.

ART algorithms can follow a person's physiological changes over time through ongoing monitoring and adaptation. Through the detection of minute changes in neuromuscular patterns or biomechanics, ART can trigger program modifications that maintain their efficacy and match the changing requirements of the individual.

This flexibility keeps performance increases from plateauing and is essential in avoiding burnout or overuse issues. When applied to long-term maintenance plans, ART increases peak performance levels' sustainability and promotes long-term success across a range of fields.

The utilization of Advanced Adaptive Resonance Theory (ART) in prehabilitation techniques, performance optimization, and long-term maintenance demonstrates the applicability of this methodology in a variety of domains. When used in sports, healthcare, or other fields, ART's adaptable character is crucial for customizing therapies to meet the needs of each patient, maximizing results, and fostering long-term well-being. A new age in individualized and anticipatory techniques is heralded by the integration of ART, which breaks through conventional paradigms to promote improved performance, injury avoidance, and long-term vitality.

CHAPTER EIGHT

STUDIES AND PROOF IN FAVOR OF ART

RESEARCH AND RESULTS FROM SCIENCE

Much scientific research has examined assisted reproductive technology (ART) to better understand its effectiveness and implications for fertility treatments. A key component of these studies concerns the success rates of several ART techniques, including intracytoplasmic sperm injection (ICSI) and in vitro fertilization (IVF).

Studies have shown time and again how effective ART is at assisting couples in overcoming infertility obstacles. For example, research frequently highlights the higher chance of live births and successful pregnancies among those receiving ART as opposed to conventional reproductive therapies.

Furthermore, studies by scientists explore the variables that affect the effectiveness of ART, such as age, underlying health issues, and the caliber of the gametes used. The aforementioned studies provide significant contributions to the enhancement of treatment protocols, patient selection criteria, and overall procedure efficiency in antiretroviral therapy. Furthermore, studies have concentrated on cutting-edge methods and technologies in the field of assisted reproductive technology (ART), including cryopreservation and preimplantation genetic testing (PGT), offering more proof of the field's ongoing development.

CRITICISMS AND DEBATES

Even though ART is widely accepted and used, disagreements and criticisms still arise in the profession. Debates within the scientific community and outside have been prompted by ethical concerns over the development and manipulation of embryos, the possibility of multiple pregnancies, and the long-term health ramifications for both mothers and progeny. The commercialization of fertility therapies, according to critics, may result in medical overuse and needless procedures, casting doubt on the social and financial implications of assisted reproductive technologies.

Disparities in access to ART therapies also give rise to controversy, with concerns about insurance coverage, pricing, and geographic differences affecting the fair distribution of reproductive healthcare.

Further adding to the current conversation in the fields of medicine, law, and ethics are the ethical issues surrounding the choice and disposal of embryos during the assisted reproductive technology (ART) procedure. The ethical quandaries surrounding assisted reproductive technologies (ART) are subject to constant discussion and adjustment in regulatory frameworks to tackle new issues as they arise.

To sum up, the scientific research substantiating ART emphasizes how well it works to treat infertility problems and increase the likelihood of a healthy pregnancy.

Nonetheless, disagreements and criticisms about moral, societal, and financial issues serve as a reminder of the necessity of applying ART with moderation and consideration, guaranteeing ethical and fair reproductive healthcare procedures.

CHAPTER NINE

EDUCATION AND ACCREDITATION IN ACTIVE RELEASE METHODS

RESOURCES FOR EDUCATION

Training in Active Release Techniques (ART) is a thorough educational process that gives medical professionals the tools they need to identify and treat soft tissue injuries. The combination of theoretical understanding and real-world, hands-on training forms the basis of an ART education. This learning process is facilitated by several materials, such as instructional films, online courses, and textbooks.

To learn about the complexities of anatomy and treatment plans, textbooks like "Active Release Techniques Soft Tissue Management System" are invaluable resources. T

These resources aid practitioners in comprehending the basic ideas of ART, which include soft tissue manipulation and assessment.

Enhancing the visual and practical parts of Art Therapy education is made possible in large part by online courses and video content. Interactive online courses offer a dynamic environment in which students can efficiently understand methods and strategies. These tools frequently have expert teachers demonstrating particular movements and procedures, enabling practitioners to see and mimic those actions.

PROCEDURE FOR CERTIFICATION

Active Release Techniques certification is an organized process that attests to a practitioner's competence in using ART principles. This procedure usually consists of multiple important phases, starting with finishing the necessary courses. Healthcare workers might have to prove they have a basic understanding of anatomy, physiology, and pertinent medical procedures before they can apply for certification.

Practitioners can participate in ART courses to study the nuances of soft tissue manipulation and treatment after fulfilling these prerequisites. These classes provide a comprehensive approach to learning by combining both theoretical and practical components. During these workshops, participants' practical assessments gauge how well they can utilize ART techniques.

Upon finishing the necessary curriculum, candidates usually take a certification exam. This test evaluates their understanding of ART concepts, diagnostic abilities, and real-world applicability. The achievement of ART certification, which denotes a practitioner's proficiency in applying ART for the treatment of soft tissue injuries, is contingent upon passing the certification exam.

OPPORTUNITIES FOR CONTINUING EDUCATION

For practitioners of Active Release Techniques to stay current with industry innovations and develop their abilities over time, continuing education is essential.

ART encourages certified professionals to pursue continual development by providing a range of alternatives for continuing education.

In ART, advanced courses and workshops are the main means of ongoing education. These specialist courses explore cutting-edge methods, fresh insights from research, and hot topics in soft tissue care. By taking part in these programs, practitioners can broaden their scope of practice and enhance their level of skill.

Additionally, seminars and conferences give ART practitioners a forum for networking and knowledge sharing. Expert speakers, case studies, and discussions of recent advances in the subject are frequently featured at these gatherings.

Participation in these events promotes a culture of continuous improvement and builds a sense of community among practitioners.

To keep their certification, practitioners usually need to take part in continuing education, which makes sure they stay up to date on the most recent developments and uphold the highest standards of Active Release Techniques practice. Maintaining the highest standard of care for patients and being at the forefront of the management of soft tissue injuries depends on this dedication to lifelong learning.

CHAPTER TEN

UPCOMING DEVELOPMENTS AND TRENDS

NEW DEVELOPMENTS IN SOFT TISSUE TREATMENTS

With the emergence of new technology in soft tissue therapy, tremendous progress is being achieved in the field of healthcare. Using cutting-edge imaging methods to improve diagnosis and treatment planning, such as magnetic resonance elastography and high-resolution ultrasound, is one notable breakthrough. With the use of these technologies, physicians can now treat patients with greater precision and focus thanks to their unparalleled understanding of soft tissue architecture.

Furthermore, the field of customized medicine is changing as a result of the incorporation of artificial intelligence (AI) in soft tissue therapies. Large-scale datasets are analyzed by AI algorithms to find trends and connections, which help with the creation of personalized treatment regimens for each patient. This is a major advancement in patient-centered care as it not only increases the effectiveness of interventions but also reduces the possibility of negative side effects.

The emergence of regenerative medicine in soft tissue therapies is another encouraging development. To replace and repair damaged tissues, stem cell therapies and tissue engineering approaches are being investigated. This could lead to a paradigm shift in the way injuries and degenerative diseases are treated. These regenerative methods have the potential to improve afflicted tissues' normal function in addition to relieving symptoms.

In addition, the incorporation of telehealth platforms into soft tissue therapies is improving service continuity and accessibility. Real-time tracking of patient progress is made possible by wearable technology, virtual consultations, and remote monitoring, which allows for prompt modifications to treatment regimens.

The traditional patient-doctor connection is being transformed by this integrated approach, which is also encouraging a more proactive and collaborative healthcare model.

CHANGING REHABILITATION PRACTICES

As the area of rehabilitation undergoes profound transformations, the way that functional abilities are restored and enhanced is being redefined through developing practices. The growing focus on individualized and patient-centered rehabilitation programs is one noteworthy trend. Modern evaluation instruments, such as wearable technology and motion capture, enable therapists to customize treatments according to each patient's needs and development, improving results and lowering the chance of relapse.

Both augmented reality (AR) and virtual reality (VR) are becoming more and more effective instruments in rehabilitation procedures. With the help of these technologies, patients can enhance their motor skills, cognitive function, and overall rehabilitation progress in a controlled yet difficult environment that simulates real-world events. In addition to adding interest to rehabilitation, VR and AR also improve neuroplasticity, which helps patients recover more quickly.

Rehabilitation techniques are increasingly embracing collaborative and multidisciplinary approaches. A thorough and all-encompassing rehabilitation experience is guaranteed by combining the knowledge of multiple healthcare professionals, such as psychologists, dietitians, occupational therapists, and physiotherapists. This multimodal approach promotes total well-being by taking into account the psychological and social aspects of rehabilitation in addition to the physical aspects.

Additionally, the field of physical therapy is changing as a result of the incorporation of robotics in rehabilitation. Individuals with mobility disabilities can benefit from precise and focused support from robotic exoskeletons and assistive devices, which can enhance their freedom and quality of life. These developments in technology support patients on their path to recovery while also enhancing the capacities of rehabilitation specialists.

The field of soft tissue therapies and rehabilitation is changing as a result of the convergence of cutting-edge technologies and changing practices. These developments represent a paradigm shift toward more efficient, patient-centric, and interdisciplinary approaches in healthcare, from tailored interventions and immersive technologies in rehabilitation to enhanced diagnostics and regenerative medicine in soft tissue therapies.

www.ingramcontent.com/pod-product-compliance
Lightning Source LLC
Chambersburg PA
CBHW070336290526
45791CB00003B/1353